The Comple

User Handbook

Safe Use, Dosage Guidelines, Side Effects,

and Interactions Explained Clearly

Dr. Fred Lanks

Table of Contents

Chapter 1: Understanding Advil

What Is Advil?

Advil is a brand name for a medicine called **ibuprofen**, which is a type of drug known as a **nonsteroidal anti-inflammatory drug (NSAID)**. It's one of the most common over-the-counter (OTC) medications used to relieve **pain, reduce inflammation, and bring down fevers**. You can buy Advil at just about any pharmacy or grocery store without a prescription, although stronger doses are available through a doctor.

People use Advil for many reasons—headaches, muscle aches, menstrual cramps, toothaches, back pain, arthritis, and more. It's also helpful for bringing down a fever, whether it's from the flu, an infection, or another illness. What makes Advil especially popular is that it works fairly quickly and doesn't cause drowsiness like some other pain medications.

While Advil is safe when used correctly, it's still a powerful drug. It's not just a simple painkiller—it affects how your body responds to pain and swelling. That's why it's important to know how it works, how much to take, and when not to use it. Understanding Advil can help you get the relief you need without running into problems.

How Advil Works in the Body

To understand how Advil helps with pain and inflammation, it helps to know what happens in your body when something goes wrong—like when you get hurt or sick. Your body produces natural chemicals called **prostaglandins**. These chemicals cause **pain, swelling, and fever** as part of your body's healing response.

Advil (ibuprofen) works by **blocking an enzyme** called **cyclooxygenase (COX)**, which your body needs to make prostaglandins. When Advil blocks this enzyme, it **lowers the amount of prostaglandins**, which in turn **reduces pain, swelling, and fever**. It doesn't fix the problem causing the pain, but it makes you feel better while your body heals.

The effects of Advil usually begin within **30 minutes to an hour** after taking it, and the relief can last about **4 to 6 hours**. That's why people often take it multiple times a day, depending on their condition.

It's important to take Advil with food or milk to protect your stomach. Because it reduces prostaglandins—and those also help protect the stomach lining—taking Advil on an empty stomach can sometimes cause irritation or ulcers. So even though Advil works well, it's best to use it wisely.

Forms and Strengths Available

Advil comes in **several forms and strengths**, making it easier for people to take it in the way that works best for them. The most common form is the **coated tablet**, but you can also find **capsules, gel capsules (called Liqui-Gels), chewable tablets, and oral suspensions (liquids)** for children. Each form is made for different needs and age groups.

For adults, the standard over-the-counter strength is **200 milligrams (mg)** per tablet or capsule. Most people take **one or two pills every 4 to 6 hours**, but shouldn't take more than **1,200 mg in a single day** unless a doctor says otherwise. Prescription-strength ibuprofen can go up to **400 mg, 600 mg, or even 800 mg per dose**, and should only be used under medical supervision.

For children, Advil comes in **liquid form** with dosing based on the child's **weight and age**. There are also **chewable tablets** made for older children who may not like swallowing pills.

There are also **combination products**, like Advil PM, which includes a sleep aid, and Advil Cold & Sinus, which includes ingredients for cold symptoms. When choosing a product, it's important to read the label carefully to make sure you're getting the right type and strength for your needs.

Chapter 2: Proper Dosage and Administration

Recommended Dosages for Adults and Children

Advil (ibuprofen) is a common over-the-counter medication used to relieve pain, reduce inflammation, and lower fever. However, taking the correct dose is very important for safety and effectiveness.

For **adults and teenagers (12 years and older)**, the typical dose is **200 to 400 mg every 4 to 6 hours** as needed. You should not take more than **1,200 mg in 24 hours** unless your doctor has told you otherwise. That's usually no more than 6 regular-strength tablets a day.

For **children under 12 years**, the dosage depends on the child's **weight and age**. Children's Advil comes in liquid form, chewable tablets, and infant drops. The label includes a dosing chart to help you find the right amount. For example, a child who weighs 24–35 pounds (around 2–3 years old) might get **5 mL of liquid every 6–8 hours**, but never more than 4 doses in 24 hours.

It's very important to **use the correct measuring device** that comes with the medicine. Never guess or use a kitchen spoon. Also, never give adult-strength Advil to a child. Always follow label instructions or talk to your doctor or pharmacist.

How and When to Take Advil Safely

Taking Advil safely means knowing when to use it, how much to take, and how to avoid problems. Advil works best when taken **at the first sign of pain** or fever, whether it's from a headache, muscle ache, period cramps, backache, or minor arthritis.

You should always **take Advil with food or milk** to protect your stomach. It can irritate your stomach lining if taken on an empty stomach, especially if you use it often. Drinking a full glass of water with your dose is also a good idea.

Stick to the timing guidelines—**every 4 to 6 hours**, and don't take more than recommended. Doubling up on doses because the pain hasn't gone away can lead to **serious health issues**, like stomach bleeding or kidney damage. If pain persists, it's better to talk to your doctor rather than keep taking more pills.

Avoid mixing Advil with **alcohol** or other medications like aspirin, blood thinners, or other NSAIDs unless your doctor says it's okay. Combining drugs can increase your risk of side effects.

If you ever miss a dose and are taking Advil on a regular schedule, **take it when you remember**, but never double up to make up for a missed dose.

Adjusting Dosage for Special Populations (Elderly, Pregnant Women, etc.)

Some people need to be more cautious with Advil, especially **older adults**, **pregnant women**, and those with **certain medical conditions**.

For **elderly people**, the kidneys don't work as well as they did in younger years, and the stomach lining becomes more fragile. Because of this, they are more likely to experience side effects like bleeding, ulcers, or kidney problems. Doctors often recommend starting at the **lowest possible dose** and avoiding long-term use unless supervised. Taking it with food and plenty of fluids is especially important.

For **pregnant women**, Advil should generally be **avoided, especially during the third trimester**. It can cause problems for both the baby and the mother, including issues with fetal heart development and reduced amniotic fluid. In early pregnancy, it may increase the risk of miscarriage. If pain relief is needed, **acetaminophen (Tylenol)** is usually recommended as a safer option. Always consult your doctor before taking any medication during pregnancy.

For people with **asthma, heart disease, high blood pressure, liver, or kidney disease**, the dose may also need to be lowered or avoided altogether. These conditions can make the body more sensitive to NSAIDs like Advil.

When in doubt, talk to your doctor or pharmacist before using Advil in special situations. Your safety always comes first.

Chapter 3: Recognizing and Managing Side Effects

Common Side Effects and Their Causes

Advil (ibuprofen) is one of the most popular over-the-counter medications for pain and inflammation. While it's generally safe for most people when used correctly, it can cause some side effects—even at normal doses. The most common side effects are usually mild and temporary, but it's still important to understand them and why they happen.

One of the most frequent issues is **stomach upset**. This includes symptoms like nausea, bloating, heartburn, or mild stomach pain. This happens because Advil belongs to a group of medications called NSAIDs (non-steroidal anti-inflammatory drugs), which can irritate the stomach lining. Taking it without food or in high doses makes this worse.

Some people also experience **dizziness or headache** after taking Advil. This might occur due to changes in blood flow or sensitivity to the drug. **Ringing in the ears (tinnitus)** is another rare but possible effect with frequent use.

Other mild symptoms can include **rash, itching, or feeling tired**. These usually go away when the medicine is stopped. Even though these effects aren't dangerous, they're signs your body might not be handling the medication well. If they happen often, talk to your doctor or pharmacist.

Serious Side Effects and When to Seek Help

While most people take Advil without major problems, some may experience serious side effects that need medical attention right away. These reactions are rare but can be life-threatening if ignored.

One of the most serious risks is **stomach bleeding or ulcers**. Signs include black or bloody stools, vomiting blood (which may look like coffee grounds), or severe stomach pain. These symptoms mean you should stop using Advil and go to the emergency room immediately.

Another risk is **kidney damage**, especially in people who are dehydrated, older, or already have kidney problems. Warning signs include little or no urine, swelling in your legs or ankles, and fatigue. Don't wait—see a doctor if you notice these.

Advil can also cause **allergic reactions**, including **swelling of the face or throat, trouble breathing, or a skin rash that spreads quickly**. These are medical emergencies. Call 911 or go to the hospital right away.

In rare cases, **heart attack or stroke** has been linked to high or long-term use of ibuprofen, especially in people with existing heart conditions. Chest pain, shortness of breath, slurred speech, or weakness in one part of your body are all signs that you need help immediately.

How to Reduce Risk of Adverse Effects

The best way to stay safe while using Advil is to take a few smart precautions. Even though side effects can happen, many are preventable with the right habits.

Always take the lowest dose that helps your pain and **only for the shortest time necessary**. Long-term or high-dose use increases the chances of serious problems like ulcers, kidney damage, or heart trouble.

Take Advil with food or milk to help protect your stomach. This simple step can reduce the risk of irritation and pain. If you already have stomach problems, ask your doctor if it's safe to use at all.

Avoid combining Advil with **other NSAIDs**, such as aspirin or naproxen, unless directed by a healthcare provider. Using more than one at the same time can increase your risk of side effects, especially stomach bleeding.

Stay well-hydrated, especially if you're using Advil for several days in a row. This helps your kidneys flush the drug out properly.

Finally, **tell your doctor or pharmacist** about all other medicines, vitamins, or conditions you have. Some drugs and diseases don't mix well with Advil. Being open with your healthcare provider can help you avoid dangerous interactions or complications.

Chapter 4: Interactions with Other Medications and Conditions

Drugs That Interact with Advil

Advil, also known as ibuprofen, can interact with many other medications. These interactions can sometimes make Advil less effective or cause serious health problems. That's why it's important to talk to your doctor or pharmacist before using it if you're already on other medicines.

One major group of drugs that interact with Advil are **blood thinners**, like warfarin or aspirin. Taking them together can increase your risk of bleeding. **High blood pressure medications**—such as ACE inhibitors, diuretics, or beta-blockers—may not work as well when taken with Advil. This can raise your blood pressure or strain your kidneys.

Other NSAIDs like naproxen or celecoxib shouldn't be used with Advil either, since combining them increases the risk of stomach ulcers, bleeding, and kidney damage. **Antidepressants** such as SSRIs (like fluoxetine or sertraline) can also increase the risk of bleeding if taken with Advil.

If you're taking medications for diabetes, heart disease, arthritis, or even cold and flu, always double-check the label. Many of these products contain NSAIDs or ingredients that may not mix well with Advil. When in doubt, ask your pharmacist or doctor to review your medicine list before adding Advil.

Health Conditions Affected by Advil Use

Advil may seem like a simple pain reliever, but it can affect several health conditions. If you have certain chronic illnesses, taking Advil without guidance can lead to more problems than it solves.

People with **kidney problems** should be especially careful. Advil can reduce blood flow to the kidneys, which can worsen kidney function, especially if you're dehydrated or already dealing with kidney disease. The same goes for people with **high blood pressure or heart disease**. Advil can make these conditions worse by causing fluid retention, raising blood pressure, or increasing the risk of heart attack or stroke—especially if taken in high doses over a long time.

If you have a **history of stomach ulcers or gastrointestinal bleeding**, Advil can irritate the stomach lining and cause ulcers to return or bleed. People with **asthma** may also experience breathing issues, as Advil can sometimes trigger asthma attacks in sensitive individuals.

Those with **liver disease** need to use caution, too. While Advil isn't metabolized the same way as acetaminophen, it can still put extra stress on the liver if used excessively. Always speak with your doctor if you have any of these conditions and are thinking of using Advil regularly.

Alcohol, Supplements, and Lifestyle Factors

The way you live—what you eat, drink, and take—can affect how Advil works in your body. Let's start with **alcohol**. Drinking while taking Advil increases the risk of stomach bleeding and liver strain. Even a few drinks a day can make this risk worse, especially if you're taking Advil often or in high doses.

Supplements can also interact with Advil, even though many people assume they're harmless. For example, **ginkgo biloba**, **garlic**, **fish oil**, and **vitamin E** all have blood-thinning effects. When combined with Advil, the risk of internal bleeding increases. **St. John's Wort**, used for mood support, may reduce the effectiveness of certain medications and could have unpredictable effects when taken with pain relievers like Advil.

Your **diet** matters too. Taking Advil on an empty stomach can irritate your gut, so it's best to take it with food or milk. Also, people on low-sodium diets due to heart or kidney issues should be aware that some Advil products contain sodium.

Finally, heavy exercise, dehydration, or high heat (like saunas or hot yoga) can strain your kidneys. Since Advil also affects kidney function, it's best to avoid these stressors while using the medication. Always stay hydrated and use it wisely.

Chapter 5: Special Considerations and Warnings

Use in Pregnancy and Breastfeeding

Using Advil (ibuprofen) during pregnancy is something that should be approached with caution. In early pregnancy (first and second trimester), occasional use may be considered safe by some doctors, but it's best to avoid it unless absolutely necessary. The real concern begins in the third trimester. Taking Advil during the last three months of pregnancy can harm the baby's heart and reduce the amount of amniotic fluid around the baby. It might also delay labor or cause complications during delivery.

If you're pregnant or planning to become pregnant, it's important to talk to your doctor before taking any medication, including Advil. There may be safer alternatives like acetaminophen (Tylenol), but even those should be used under guidance.

When it comes to breastfeeding, small amounts of ibuprofen can pass into breast milk, but it's generally considered safe for nursing mothers. It's one of the preferred pain relievers during breastfeeding, especially because only tiny amounts reach the baby. Still, if your baby is premature or has other health issues, always double-check with your pediatrician.

The bottom line: Don't self-medicate during pregnancy or while breastfeeding. Always ask a healthcare provider first before taking Advil.

Children and Teen Use: What Parents Should Know

Advil can be safely used in children and teens, but only when given in the right way. It's important for parents to understand that kids are not just "small adults" — their bodies work differently, and dosages need to be based on weight, not just age. Advil makes special formulas for children (Children's Advil and Infants' Advil), which come in liquids, chewables, or drops. Always use the measuring tool provided and follow the dosage chart carefully.

Never give adult Advil to a child unless told by a doctor. Too much ibuprofen can lead to serious problems like stomach bleeding, kidney damage, or even overdose.

For teens, it's still important to monitor how much they take and how often. Some teens may try to take more than the recommended dose if they're in a lot of pain or think it will work faster. Remind them that more is not better—and that overuse can be dangerous.

Also, make sure your child or teen isn't taking multiple medications that may contain ibuprofen or other NSAIDs. Double-dosing can happen by mistake. If you're ever unsure, call a doctor or pharmacist before giving any medicine.

Long-Term Use and Potential Risks

Advil is great for short-term relief of pain, inflammation, and fever. But when it's used for a long time, especially without a doctor's supervision, problems can start to build up. Many people with chronic pain, like arthritis sufferers, might rely on Advil daily. While it can help, this kind of regular use comes with risks.

One of the biggest concerns with long-term Advil use is damage to the stomach lining. It can cause ulcers, stomach bleeding, or chronic indigestion. Taking Advil with food can help a bit, but it doesn't eliminate the risk. Using it with other NSAIDs or alcohol increases the danger.

Another serious risk is kidney damage. Over time, ibuprofen can affect how the kidneys filter blood and remove waste. People with existing kidney problems, heart issues, or high blood pressure are especially vulnerable.

There's also a risk to the heart. Studies have shown that regular, high-dose ibuprofen use might increase the risk of heart attacks and strokes, especially in older adults or those with heart disease.

To use Advil safely long-term, regular check-ups are a must. Your doctor may suggest using the lowest effective dose for the shortest time possible—or switching to other treatments.

Chapter 6: Alternatives, Overdose, and Emergency Guidance

When Not to Use Advil: Safer Alternatives

There are times when taking Advil might not be the best choice. If you have certain health conditions like stomach ulcers, kidney disease, liver problems, or a history of heart issues, it's important to avoid Advil. That's because Advil, which contains ibuprofen, can irritate the stomach lining, strain the kidneys, and increase the risk of heart problems when used too often or in high doses.

Also, if you're allergic to aspirin or other nonsteroidal anti-inflammatory drugs (NSAIDs), Advil is not safe for you. You should also avoid it before or after certain surgeries, like heart bypass surgery, unless your doctor says otherwise. Pregnant women, especially in the third trimester, should not use Advil unless told to by a healthcare provider, as it may affect the baby's heart or reduce amniotic fluid.

If Advil isn't safe for you, don't worry—there are alternatives. Acetaminophen (Tylenol) is often a gentler option, especially for pain and fever, and it's easier on the stomach. You can also consider natural remedies like applying ice, using heat pads, trying gentle stretching, or taking turmeric supplements for inflammation. Always talk to a doctor or pharmacist before switching medications to make sure it's right for you.

Signs of Overdose and Immediate Actions

Taking too much Advil, either by accident or on purpose, can lead to an overdose, which is serious and needs quick action. An overdose happens when someone takes more than the recommended dose, either at once or over time. Signs to watch for include nausea, vomiting, stomach pain, drowsiness, headache, ringing in the ears, and feeling dizzy. If the overdose is severe, symptoms can get worse and may include trouble breathing, seizures, confusion, or even fainting.

Some people might not show symptoms right away, but the damage to the kidneys, stomach, or liver could still be happening inside the body. That's why it's important not to wait for something to feel "bad" before acting.

If you think someone has taken too much Advil, call emergency services (911 in the U.S.) or your local poison control center immediately. Don't try to make the person vomit unless a medical professional tells you to. Try to keep the person calm, and if possible, tell the doctor how much Advil was taken, when it was taken, and whether it was mixed with alcohol or other drugs. Quick action can help prevent serious health problems or even save a life.

What to Do in Case of Accidental Ingestion

Accidental ingestion of Advil can happen, especially with young children, elderly people, or even pets. If someone takes Advil without meaning to—maybe a child grabs a tablet thinking it's candy, or an older adult takes an extra dose by mistake—it's important to act fast and stay calm.

The first thing to do is check how much was taken and when. For small children, even a small dose can be harmful. Symptoms to watch for include stomach pain, nausea, vomiting, sleepiness, or irritability. In serious cases, the person might have trouble breathing, look very pale, or become unresponsive.

If a child or adult has accidentally swallowed Advil, call your local poison control center right away. In the U.S., you can call 1-800-222-1222. If the person shows any serious signs, such as trouble breathing or unconsciousness, call emergency services immediately.

Do not wait for symptoms to appear before getting help. The sooner you act, the better the chances of avoiding serious problems. Also, don't give the person food, drink, or anything else unless advised by a healthcare provider. And remember, always store Advil and all medications out of reach of children and pets to help prevent these accidents in the future.

Conclusion

Key Takeaways for Safe and Effective Use

Advil is helpful when used the right way. Always read the label and follow the exact dose. Taking too much can hurt your stomach, liver, or kidneys. Don't mix it with alcohol or other medicines unless your doctor says it's okay. Take it with food or milk to avoid stomach pain. Don't use it longer than recommended without a doctor's advice. If symptoms don't improve in a few days, stop and get help. Store Advil in a cool, dry place, and keep it away from children. Being careful helps you stay safe and feel better faster.

When to Consult a Healthcare Professional

You should talk to a doctor if Advil doesn't help your pain after a few days or if the pain gets worse. If you feel dizzy, have stomach bleeding, rashes, or breathing problems, stop taking it and get medical help right away. Always check with your doctor if you're pregnant, breastfeeding, have heart, kidney, or liver problems, or are on other medications. If you're not sure whether Advil is right for you, ask your pharmacist or doctor. It's better to be safe than sorry. Never guess with your health—professionals are there to guide and protect you.

Final Thoughts on Responsible Pain Management

Pain is real, and it's okay to need relief. But managing pain responsibly means not depending on medication all the time. Advil can ease pain and swelling, but it's just one part of the solution. Try rest, gentle movement, or ice packs too. Use Advil only when necessary and not just out of habit. Always choose the lowest dose for the shortest time. Listen to your body, and don't ignore warning signs. Responsible use means knowing when to take medicine and when to explore other options. Smart choices today protect your health for the future.

Printed in Dunstable, United Kingdom